DR. BARBARA'S SIMPLE JUICE DETOX FOR OVER 50

Your step-by-step guide to obtaining optimal wellness through full body detox using delicious and healthy juice recipes and smoothies

Odesa Mulan

Table of Contents

COPYRIGHT © 2023

CHAPTER ONE

The Importance of Detoxification for Health and Well-being After 50

Introduction

Entering the fifth decade of life marks a significant milestone, often accompanied by changes in health and well-being. As individuals age, their bodies undergo various physiological alterations, including decreased metabolic efficiency and increased susceptibility to toxins. Consequently, there is a growing recognition of the importance of detoxification for maintaining optimal health and well-being, particularly after the age of 50. In this comprehensive exploration, we delve into the significance of detoxification in this demographic, elucidating its impact on overall health and offering insights into effective detoxification strategies.

Understanding Detoxification

Detoxification refers to the physiological process by which the body eliminates toxins and harmful substances, thereby safeguarding health and promoting vitality. This intricate process primarily occurs in the liver, kidneys, gastrointestinal tract, skin, and lungs, collectively known as the body's detoxification organs. The liver, in particular, plays a central role in detoxification by metabolizing toxins and converting them into water-soluble compounds for excretion.

Challenges of Detoxification After 50

As individuals age, several factors contribute to a decline in the body's detoxification capacity, rendering them more vulnerable to the adverse effects of accumulated toxins. Age-related changes in organ function, such as decreased liver enzyme activity and renal function, can impair detoxification processes. Additionally, prolonged exposure to environmental pollutants, dietary toxins, medications, and lifestyle factors further burden the body's detoxification mechanisms, exacerbating the risk of chronic diseases and accelerated aging.

Health Implications of Toxin Accumulation

The accumulation of toxins in the body can have profound implications for health and well-being, particularly in individuals over 50. Chronic exposure to environmental toxins, such as heavy metals, pesticides, and air pollutants, has been linked to various adverse health outcomes, including cardiovascular disease, neurodegenerative disorders, cancer, and metabolic dysfunction. Furthermore, the accumulation of endogenous toxins, such as metabolic waste products and free radicals, can contribute to oxidative stress, inflammation, and cellular damage, accelerating the aging process and predisposing individuals to age-related diseases.

Benefits of Detoxification After 50

Given the deleterious effects of toxin accumulation on health, prioritizing detoxification becomes paramount, especially for individuals over 50. Effective detoxification interventions can help mitigate the burden of toxins on the body and promote overall health and vitality. By supporting the body's natural detoxification processes, individuals can enhance organ function, bolster immunity, optimize metabolic function, and mitigate the risk of chronic diseases associated with toxin exposure.

Strategies for Effective Detoxification

Several strategies can facilitate effective detoxification in individuals over 50, empowering them to safeguard their health and well-being. Dietary interventions, such as consuming a nutrient-dense, plant-based diet rich in antioxidants, fiber, and phytonutrients, can support liver function and promote toxin elimination. Hydration is also critical for detoxification, as adequate water intake facilitates the flushing of toxins from the body via the kidneys and skin.

In addition to dietary modifications, lifestyle factors play a pivotal role in detoxification. Regular physical activity enhances circulation, lymphatic drainage, and sweat production, facilitating the elimination of toxins through the skin. Moreover, stress management techniques, such as meditation, yoga, and deep breathing exercises, can mitigate the impact of psychological stress on detoxification pathways, promoting overall well-being.

Supplementation and Detoxification Protocols

Supplementation with targeted nutrients and botanicals can complement dietary and lifestyle interventions to support detoxification in individuals over 50. Key nutrients such as glutathione, N-acetylcysteine (NAC), alpha-lipoic acid, and vitamins C and E serve as cofactors for detoxification enzymes and antioxidants, aiding in toxin metabolism and neutralization. Herbal remedies such as milk thistle, dandelion root, and turmeric exhibit hepatoprotective properties and can enhance liver function and bile production, facilitating toxin elimination.

Detoxification protocols, such as intermittent fasting, juice cleanses, and sauna therapy, have gained popularity for their purported ability to promote detoxification and rejuvenate the body. However, it is essential to approach such protocols with caution, as they may not be suitable for everyone and could potentially exacerbate underlying health conditions. Consulting with a qualified healthcare practitioner before embarking on a detoxification regimen is advisable to ensure safety and efficacy.

Conclusion

In conclusion, detoxification plays a pivotal role in promoting health and well-being, particularly for individuals over 50 who may be more susceptible to the adverse effects of toxin accumulation. By supporting the body's natural detoxification processes through dietary modifications, lifestyle interventions, supplementation, and detoxification protocols, individuals can optimize organ function, mitigate the risk of chronic diseases, and enhance overall vitality. Prioritizing detoxification as part of a comprehensive approach to health maintenance is essential for thriving in the golden years and enjoying a fulfilling and active lifestyle.

CHAPTER TWO

Understanding the Aging Process: How Detox Can Support Overall Health

Introduction

Aging is a natural and inevitable process characterized by a gradual decline in physiological function and an increased susceptibility to age-related diseases. While aging is influenced by a complex interplay of genetic, environmental, and lifestyle factors, one key aspect that emerges is the accumulation of toxins and metabolic waste products in the body over time. As individuals age, their ability to effectively detoxify and eliminate these harmful substances diminishes, leading to a buildup of toxins that can contribute to the aging process and compromise overall health. In this exploration, we delve into the aging process, elucidate the role of detoxification in supporting overall health, and discuss strategies to promote effective detoxification as a means of enhancing well-being throughout the aging journey.

The Aging Process: A Complex Interplay of Factors

Aging is a multifaceted process influenced by a myriad of factors, including genetics, lifestyle choices, environmental exposures, and physiological changes. At the cellular level, aging is characterized by a progressive decline in cellular function and integrity, accompanied by an accumulation of cellular damage and alterations in gene expression. Key hallmarks of aging include genomic instability, telomere attrition, epigenetic alterations, mitochondrial dysfunction, and cellular senescence, all of which contribute to the overall aging phenotype.

In addition to cellular changes, aging is also associated with alterations in tissue structure and function, including loss of muscle mass and strength, decreased bone density, impaired immune function, and diminished organ reserve. These physiological changes predispose individuals to age-related diseases such as cardiovascular disease, neurodegenerative disorders, cancer, and metabolic dysfunction, ultimately impacting quality of life and longevity.

The Role of Toxins in Aging

Toxins are ubiquitous in the modern environment, encompassing a wide range of exogenous and endogenous substances that can adversely affect health. Exogenous toxins include environmental pollutants, heavy metals, pesticides, pharmaceutical drugs, and food additives, while endogenous toxins refer to metabolic byproducts such as reactive oxygen species (ROS) and advanced glycation end-products (AGEs). Both exogenous and endogenous toxins can accumulate in the body over time, overwhelming the body's detoxification systems and contributing to the aging process.

The accumulation of toxins in various tissues and organs can disrupt cellular function, impair mitochondrial activity, promote oxidative stress and inflammation, and accelerate cellular aging. Furthermore, toxins can interfere with cellular signaling pathways, disrupt hormone balance, and compromise immune function, predisposing individuals to a wide range of age-related diseases and health conditions.

Detoxification: A Vital Process for Health and Longevity

Detoxification is the body's natural process of eliminating toxins and harmful substances to maintain internal balance and promote optimal health. The liver, kidneys, gastrointestinal tract, skin, and lungs are the primary organs involved in detoxification, each playing a distinct role in the elimination of toxins from the body. The liver, in particular, serves as the body's primary detoxification organ, where toxins are metabolized, conjugated, and excreted via bile or urine.

Effective detoxification is essential for supporting overall health and longevity, as it helps prevent the accumulation of toxins and reduces the burden on the body's detoxification systems. By promoting optimal liver function, enhancing antioxidant defenses, and supporting the elimination of toxins through various pathways, detoxification can mitigate the risk of age-related diseases, improve cellular function, and promote vitality throughout the aging process.

Strategies to Support Detoxification and Enhance Overall Health

Several strategies can help support detoxification and enhance overall health, particularly as individuals age and face increased challenges in eliminating toxins from the body. Dietary interventions, such as consuming a nutrient-dense, plant-based diet rich in antioxidants, fiber, and phytonutrients, can support liver function and promote the elimination of toxins through the gastrointestinal tract.

Hydration is also critical for detoxification, as adequate water intake supports kidney function and facilitates the excretion of toxins via urine. Additionally, regular physical activity promotes lymphatic drainage, circulation, and sweat production, aiding in the elimination of toxins through the skin. Stress management techniques, such as meditation, yoga, and deep breathing exercises, can help mitigate the impact of psychological stress on detoxification pathways, promoting overall well-being.

Supplementation with targeted nutrients and botanicals can complement dietary and lifestyle interventions to support detoxification and enhance overall health. Key nutrients such as glutathione, N-acetylcysteine (NAC), alpha-lipoic acid, and vitamins C and E serve as cofactors for detoxification enzymes and antioxidants, aiding in toxin metabolism and neutralization. Herbal remedies such as milk thistle, dandelion root, and turmeric exhibit hepatoprotective properties and can enhance liver function, facilitating toxin elimination.

Conclusion

In conclusion, the aging process is characterized by a complex interplay of genetic, environmental, and lifestyle factors that contribute to cellular dysfunction, tissue damage, and increased susceptibility to age-related diseases. The accumulation of toxins in the body plays a significant role in the aging process, disrupting cellular function, promoting oxidative stress and inflammation, and compromising overall health and longevity. Effective detoxification is essential for supporting overall health and vitality throughout the aging journey, as it helps prevent the buildup of toxins and reduces the burden on the body's detoxification systems. By implementing dietary, lifestyle, and supplementation strategies to support detoxification, individuals can enhance overall health, mitigate the risk of age-related diseases, and promote vitality and longevity as they age.

CHAPTER THREE

Preparing for a Juice Detox: Safety Considerations and Precautions

Embarking on a juice detox can be a rejuvenating experience for many, offering a chance to reset dietary habits, flush out toxins, and revitalize the body. However, like any significant dietary change or cleanse, it's essential to approach a juice detox with caution and consideration for safety. In this guide, we'll explore the key safety considerations and precautions to take when preparing for a juice detox, ensuring a safe and beneficial experience.

Understanding Juice Detox

A juice detox, also known as a juice cleanse or juice fast, typically involves consuming only fresh fruit and vegetable juices for a specified period, ranging from a few days to several weeks. Proponents of juice detoxes claim various health benefits, including improved digestion, increased energy, weight loss, and detoxification of the body.

Consultation with Healthcare Professional

Before starting any detoxification program, including a juice cleanse, it's crucial to consult with a healthcare professional, especially if you have any underlying health conditions or concerns. A qualified healthcare provider can assess your individual health status, provide personalized recommendations, and ensure that a juice detox is safe and appropriate for you.

Considerations for Certain Health Conditions

Individuals with certain health conditions may need to exercise caution or avoid juice detoxes altogether. For example, individuals with diabetes should closely monitor their blood sugar levels during a juice cleanse, as fruit juices can contain high amounts of natural sugars that may affect blood glucose levels. Similarly, individuals with kidney disease may need to limit their intake of potassium-rich juices, such as orange or tomato juice, to avoid putting additional strain on the kidneys.

Gradual Transition and Preparation

Rather than jumping straight into a juice detox, it's advisable to gradually transition your diet in the days leading up to the cleanse. Start by eliminating processed foods, caffeine, alcohol, and refined sugars from your diet and increasing your intake of fruits, vegetables, and whole grains. This gradual transition can help reduce withdrawal symptoms and prepare your body for the detoxification process.

Hydration and Nutrient Intake

While juice detoxes can provide a concentrated source of vitamins, minerals, and antioxidants, they may lack essential nutrients such as protein, fiber, and healthy fats. It's essential to stay adequately hydrated during a juice cleanse by drinking plenty of water throughout the day. Additionally, consider incorporating vegetable juices that contain leafy greens, such as kale or spinach, to boost your intake of fiber and micronutrients.

Listen to Your Body

During a juice detox, pay close attention to how your body responds and adjust your approach accordingly. If you experience symptoms such as dizziness, fatigue, headaches, or nausea, it may be a sign that the detoxification process is too intense or that your body needs additional support. Consider incorporating small meals or snacks, such as raw fruits or vegetables, to provide extra energy and nutrients as needed.

Duration and Frequency

The duration and frequency of a juice detox can vary depending on individual goals and preferences. While some people may choose to do a short-term cleanse lasting one to three days, others may opt for longer cleanses lasting one to two weeks. It's essential to listen to your body and avoid prolonged or excessively restrictive detoxes that could potentially compromise your health.

Post-Detox Transition

After completing a juice detox, gradually reintroduce solid foods into your diet to prevent digestive discomfort and support long-term dietary habits. Start with easily digestible foods such as steamed vegetables, soups, and whole grains, and gradually reintroduce other foods over the course of several days. Pay attention to how your body responds to different foods and make adjustments as needed to maintain the benefits of the detox.

Conclusion

In conclusion, while a juice detox can offer many potential health benefits, it's essential to approach it with caution and consideration for safety. Consulting with a healthcare professional, gradual transition and preparation, staying hydrated, listening to your body, and following appropriate duration and frequency guidelines are key steps to ensure a safe and beneficial juice detox experience. By taking these precautions and incorporating healthy lifestyle habits, you can maximize the benefits of a juice detox while safeguarding your overall health and well-being.

CHAPTER FOUR

Introduction to Herbal Juicing for Detoxification

Welcome to Day 1 of your journey into herbal juicing for detoxification! Herbal juicing offers a natural and effective way to support your body's detoxification processes, promoting vitality and well-being. In this introductory guide, we'll explore the fundamentals of herbal juicing for detoxification, including the benefits of herbal ingredients, tips for selecting and preparing herbs, and simple recipes to kick-start your detox journey.

Understanding Herbal Juicing for Detoxification

Herbal juicing involves extracting the nutrients and beneficial compounds from various herbs and incorporating them into fresh fruit and vegetable juices. Herbs are prized for their potent medicinal properties, including detoxifying, anti-inflammatory, and antioxidant effects, making them valuable additions to any detox regimen.

Benefits of Herbal Ingredients

Herbs contain a wide array of bioactive compounds, including vitamins, minerals, antioxidants, and phytochemicals, that support detoxification and overall health. For example, dandelion root is renowned for its liver-cleansing properties, while parsley acts as a natural diuretic, aiding in the elimination of toxins through the urinary system. Other herbs such as cilantro, ginger, and turmeric possess anti-inflammatory and antioxidant properties that help combat oxidative stress and support cellular health.

Selecting and Preparing Herbal Ingredients

When selecting herbs for juicing, opt for fresh, organic varieties whenever possible to ensure optimal quality and potency. Wash herbs thoroughly to remove any dirt or residue, and remove any tough stems or woody parts before juicing. Experiment with a variety of herbs to discover your preferred flavor combinations and therapeutic effects.

Simple Herbal Juice Recipes

To get you started on your herbal juicing journey, here are two simple and refreshing juice recipes featuring detoxifying herbs:

1. **Liver Cleanse Juice**

    - Ingredients:

        - 1 medium beetroot

        - 2 carrots

        - 1 cucumber

        - 1-inch piece of ginger

        - Handful of fresh dandelion leaves

- Directions:

1. Wash and chop all ingredients into manageable pieces.

2. Pass the ingredients through a juicer, alternating between firmer and softer ingredients to ensure efficient juicing.

3. Stir the juice well and serve immediately over ice, if desired.

2. **Green Detox Juice**

- Ingredients:

    - 2 cups spinach

    - 1 cucumber

    - 1 green apple

    - 1 lemon (peeled)

    - Small handful of fresh parsley

- Directions:

1. Wash and prepare all ingredients as needed.

2. Juice the spinach, cucumber, green apple, lemon, and parsley using a juicer.

3. Once juiced, stir the mixture well and pour into glasses. Enjoy immediately for maximum freshness and flavor.

Tips for a Successful Herbal Juice Detox

- Stay hydrated: In addition to herbal juices, drink plenty of water throughout the day to support detoxification and hydration.

- Listen to your body: Pay attention to how your body responds to different herbs and adjust your juicing recipes accordingly.

- Incorporate other detoxifying practices: Enhance the effects of herbal juicing by incorporating other detoxifying practices such as dry brushing, sauna sessions, or herbal teas.

Conclusion

Herbal juicing offers a delightful and effective way to support detoxification and promote overall health and vitality. By harnessing the power of detoxifying herbs in your juice recipes, you can enhance the benefits of your detox regimen and embark on a journey toward greater well-being. Experiment with different herbs, flavors, and combinations to discover the perfect herbal juices for your detoxification goals. Stay tuned for Day 2, where we'll delve deeper into specific herbs and their detoxifying properties. Happy juicing!

CHAPTER FIVE

Day 2: Herbal Juice Recipes to Support Digestive Health and Detoxification

Welcome to Day 2 of your herbal juicing journey! Today, we'll explore herbal juice recipes specifically designed to support digestive health and enhance detoxification. A healthy digestive system is essential for optimal nutrient absorption and toxin elimination, making these recipes valuable additions to your detox regimen. Let's dive into the world of digestive-supportive herbs and refreshing juice blends!

Understanding Digestive-Supportive Herbs

Certain herbs possess unique properties that can help soothe digestive discomfort, promote gut health, and support detoxification. These herbs often have carminative, anti-inflammatory, or antimicrobial properties that aid in digestion and alleviate digestive issues such as bloating, gas, and indigestion. Incorporating these herbs into your juice recipes can enhance their digestive benefits and contribute to overall well-being.

Digestive-Supportive Herbal Juice Recipes

1. **Ginger Lemon Digestive Tonic**

   - Ingredients:

- 1-inch piece of fresh ginger

- 1 lemon (peeled)

- 2 medium carrots

- 1 cucumber

- Small handful of fresh mint leaves

- Directions:

1. Wash and prepare all ingredients as needed.

2. Pass the ginger, lemon, carrots, cucumber, and mint through a juicer.

3. Stir the juice well and pour into glasses over ice, if desired. Enjoy immediately to reap the digestive benefits of ginger and lemon.

2. Pineapple Papaya Digestive Delight

- Ingredients:

- 1 cup fresh pineapple chunks

- 1 cup fresh papaya chunks

- 1 small cucumber

- Small handful of fresh basil leaves

- Directions:

1.   Wash and chop all ingredients into manageable pieces.

2.   Juice the pineapple, papaya, cucumber, and basil using a juicer.

3.   Once juiced, stir the mixture well and pour into glasses. Sip slowly and savor the tropical flavors while supporting digestive health.

Tips for Enhancing Digestive Health

- **Include fiber-rich ingredients:** Incorporate fiber-rich fruits and vegetables such as apples, pears, and leafy greens into your juice recipes to support healthy digestion and regular bowel movements.

- **Add probiotic-rich ingredients:** Consider adding probiotic-rich ingredients such as kefir, yogurt, or fermented vegetables to your juices to promote a healthy balance of gut bacteria and support digestive function.

- **Stay hydrated:** Drink plenty of water throughout the day to help flush toxins from your system and keep your digestive tract hydrated and functioning optimally.

Conclusion

These herbal juice recipes offer delicious and effective ways to support digestive health and enhance detoxification. By incorporating digestive-supportive herbs and ingredients into your juice blends, you can promote optimal digestion, alleviate digestive discomfort, and support overall well-being. Experiment with different combinations of herbs and flavors to discover the perfect juices for your digestive health goals. Stay tuned for Day 3, where we'll explore herbal juice recipes to promote immune support and vitality. Cheers to your health and happy juicing!

CHAPTER SIX

Day 3: Incorporating Nutrient-Rich Herbs into Your Detox Routine

Welcome to Day 3 of your herbal juicing adventure! Today, we'll explore the incorporation of nutrient-rich herbs into your detox routine. These herbs are powerhouses of vitamins, minerals, antioxidants, and phytonutrients, offering a potent boost to your overall health and vitality. Let's delve into some herbal juice recipes featuring nutrient-rich herbs to supercharge your detox journey.

Understanding Nutrient-Rich Herbs

Nutrient-rich herbs are abundant sources of essential vitamins, minerals, and other bioactive compounds that support various aspects of health and well-being. Incorporating these herbs into your juice recipes can help ensure that you're receiving a concentrated dose of nutrients to fuel your body and support detoxification. From leafy greens to medicinal roots, nutrient-rich herbs offer a diverse array of flavors and health benefits to explore.

Nutrient-Rich Herbal Juice Recipes

1. **Kale Spinach Super Green Juice**

    - Ingredients:

- 2 cups kale leaves

- 2 cups spinach leaves

- 1 cucumber

- 2 green apples

- 1 lemon (peeled)

- Small handful of fresh parsley

- Directions:

1. Wash and prepare all ingredients as needed.

2. Juice the kale, spinach, cucumber, green apples, lemon, and parsley using a juicer.

3. Stir the juice well and pour into glasses. Sip and enjoy the vibrant green goodness of this nutrient-rich herbal juice.

2. Turmeric Carrot Immune Booster

- Ingredients:

  - 2 large carrots

  - 1-inch piece of fresh turmeric root (or 1 teaspoon ground turmeric)

  - 1 orange (peeled)

  - 1-inch piece of ginger

- Small handful of fresh cilantro

- Directions:

1. Wash and chop all ingredients into manageable pieces.

2. Juice the carrots, turmeric, orange, and ginger using a juicer.

3. Once juiced, stir the mixture well and pour into glasses. Savor the vibrant color and immune-boosting benefits of this herbal juice blend.

Tips for Incorporating Nutrient-Rich Herbs

- **Rotate your herbs:** Experiment with a variety of nutrient-rich herbs to ensure you're receiving a diverse range of nutrients and health benefits.

- **Use organic herbs:** Whenever possible, choose organic herbs to minimize exposure to pesticides and maximize nutrient content.

- **Combine herbs with complementary ingredients:** Pair nutrient-rich herbs with fruits, vegetables, and other ingredients that complement their flavors and enhance their nutritional profile.

Conclusion

Incorporating nutrient-rich herbs into your detox routine is a delicious and effective way to support overall health and vitality.

By harnessing the power of these herbs in your juice recipes, you can ensure that you're providing your body with the essential nutrients it needs to thrive. Experiment with different combinations of herbs and ingredients to create personalized herbal juices that nourish and energize you from the inside out. Stay tuned for Day 4, where we'll explore herbal juice recipes to promote hydration and skin health. Keep juicing and enjoy the benefits of herbal nutrition!

CHAPTER SEVEN

Day 4: Herbal Supplements and Additives to Enhance Detox Results

Welcome to Day 4 of your herbal juicing journey! Today, we'll explore the use of herbal supplements and additives to enhance the results of your detoxification efforts. While herbal juices provide a potent source of nutrients and antioxidants, incorporating certain herbal supplements and additives can further support detoxification, promote vitality, and optimize overall health. Let's delve into some herbal supplements and additives to supercharge your detox routine.

Understanding Herbal Supplements and Additives

Herbal supplements and additives are natural substances derived from plants that offer specific health benefits when incorporated into your diet or wellness routine. These supplements may come in various forms, including powders, capsules, extracts, and tinctures, and can be easily integrated into your herbal juice recipes to enhance their detoxifying properties. From adaptogenic herbs to superfood powders, herbal supplements and additives offer a convenient way to boost the nutritional content and efficacy of your detox regimen.

Herbal Supplements and Additives for Detoxification

1. **Spirulina:** Spirulina is a nutrient-dense blue-green algae that is rich in protein, vitamins, minerals, and antioxidants. Adding spirulina powder to your herbal juices can support detoxification, boost energy levels, and promote overall well-being.

2. **Chlorella:** Chlorella is a freshwater algae known for its detoxifying properties. Rich in chlorophyll, vitamins, minerals, and antioxidants, chlorella helps support liver function, remove heavy metals from the body, and enhance cellular detoxification.

3. **Ashwagandha:** Ashwagandha is an adaptogenic herb that helps the body adapt to stress and promote balance. Adding ashwagandha powder to your herbal juices can support adrenal health, reduce stress levels, and enhance overall resilience during detoxification.

4. **Milk Thistle:** Milk thistle is a flowering herb traditionally used to support liver health and detoxification. Its active compound, silymarin, helps protect the liver from toxins and oxidative damage, making it a valuable addition to any detox regimen.

5. **Psyllium Husk:** Psyllium husk is a soluble fiber derived from the seeds of the Plantago ovata plant. Adding psyllium husk powder to your herbal juices can support digestive health, promote regularity, and aid in the elimination of toxins from the body.

Incorporating Herbal Supplements and Additives

To incorporate herbal supplements and additives into your detox routine, simply add the desired amount to your herbal juice recipes and blend well to combine. Start with small amounts and gradually increase as needed to achieve your desired results. Be sure to follow the recommended dosage instructions provided on the product packaging or consult with a healthcare professional for personalized guidance.

Conclusion

Herbal supplements and additives offer a convenient and effective way to enhance the results of your detoxification efforts. By incorporating nutrient-rich herbs such as spirulina, chlorella, ashwagandha, milk thistle, and psyllium husk into your herbal juices, you can support detoxification, promote vitality, and optimize overall health and well-being. Experiment with different herbal supplements and additives to discover the perfect combination for your detox routine, and enjoy the benefits of herbal nutrition. Stay tuned for Day 5, where we'll explore herbal juice recipes for relaxation and stress relief. Keep juicing and thriving on your detox journey!

CHAPTER EIGHT

Day 5: Managing Detox Symptoms and Supporting Energy Levels

Congratulations on reaching Day 5 of your herbal juicing journey! As you continue your detoxification process, it's essential to be mindful of potential detox symptoms and to support your energy levels throughout the process. In today's guide, we'll explore strategies for managing detox symptoms and maintaining optimal energy levels to ensure a successful and enjoyable detox experience.

Understanding Detox Symptoms

Detoxification can sometimes elicit temporary symptoms as your body releases toxins and adjusts to dietary changes. These symptoms may include headaches, fatigue, digestive discomfort, mood swings, and skin breakouts. While detox symptoms are often a sign that your body is cleansing and rebalancing, they can be uncomfortable to experience. Fortunately, there are several strategies you can employ to manage detox symptoms effectively.

Strategies for Managing Detox Symptoms

1. **Stay Hydrated:** Proper hydration is essential for supporting detoxification and minimizing detox symptoms. Drink plenty of water throughout the day to help flush toxins from your system and keep your body hydrated.

2. **Support Liver Function:** The liver plays a central role in detoxification, so it's crucial to support its function during a detox. Incorporate liver-supportive herbs such as dandelion root, milk thistle, and turmeric into your herbal juices to promote optimal liver function.

3. **Get Plenty of Rest:** Detoxification can be taxing on the body, so be sure to prioritize rest and relaxation during your detox journey. Aim for at least 7-8 hours of sleep per night to support your body's natural healing processes.

4. **Practice Gentle Exercise:** Engage in gentle exercise such as walking, yoga, or tai chi to support circulation, lymphatic drainage, and toxin elimination. Avoid intense workouts that may further stress your body during the detox process.

5. **Incorporate Stress Management Techniques:** Chronic stress can impair detoxification and exacerbate detox symptoms. Practice stress management techniques such as meditation, deep breathing exercises, or journaling to promote relaxation and emotional well-being.

Supporting Energy Levels

Maintaining energy levels is essential during a detox to support overall well-being and prevent fatigue. Here are some strategies to help you sustain energy levels throughout your detox journey:

1. **Include Protein and Healthy Fats:** Incorporate protein-rich ingredients such as nuts, seeds, and plant-based protein powders into your herbal juices to help stabilize blood sugar levels and sustain energy throughout the day. Adding healthy fats from sources such as avocados, coconut oil, and flaxseeds can also provide a sustained source of energy.

2. **Choose Nutrient-Dense Ingredients:**Opt for nutrient-dense fruits, vegetables, and herbs in your juice recipes to ensure you're receiving a wide array of vitamins, minerals, and antioxidants to support energy production and overall vitality.

3. **Stay Balanced:** While detoxification is beneficial, it's essential to maintain balance and avoid overly restrictive diets that may leave you feeling depleted. Listen to your body's hunger and fullness cues, and eat regular meals and snacks as needed to support energy levels.

4. **Stay Hydrated:** Dehydration can lead to feelings of fatigue and lethargy, so be sure to drink plenty of water and hydrating herbal teas throughout the day to support energy levels and overall well-being.

Conclusion

By implementing these strategies for managing detox symptoms and supporting energy levels, you can ensure a successful and enjoyable detox experience. Remember to listen to your body, prioritize rest and relaxation, and nourish yourself with nutrient-rich herbal juices and whole foods throughout your detox journey. Stay tuned for more tips and inspiration on your path to wellness. Keep juicing and thriving!

CHAPTER NINE

Day 6: Mindfulness and Relaxation Techniques for Detoxification

As you continue your herbal juicing journey, it's essential to incorporate mindfulness and relaxation techniques to support your body's detoxification process fully. Stress reduction and mental well-being are integral components of a successful detox, as they promote balance and harmony within the body. In today's guide, we'll explore mindfulness and relaxation techniques that complement your detoxification efforts, fostering a sense of calm and rejuvenation.

Understanding the Importance of Mindfulness and Relaxation

Mindfulness and relaxation techniques can help reduce stress levels, support emotional well-being, and enhance the body's natural detoxification processes. Chronic stress can impair detoxification pathways, disrupt hormonal balance, and contribute to inflammation and oxidative stress. By incorporating mindfulness and relaxation practices into your daily routine, you can create a supportive environment for detoxification and promote overall health and vitality.

Mindfulness and Relaxation Techniques for Detoxification

1. **Meditation:** Meditation is a powerful practice for calming the mind, reducing stress, and promoting relaxation. Set aside time each day for meditation, focusing on deep breathing, body scanning, or guided visualization to quiet the mind and cultivate inner peace.

2. **Yoga:** Yoga combines physical postures, breathwork, and meditation to promote relaxation, flexibility, and mental clarity. Incorporate gentle yoga sessions into your routine to release tension, improve circulation, and support detoxification through movement and breath.

3. **Deep Breathing Exercises:** Deep breathing exercises, such as diaphragmatic breathing or alternate nostril breathing, can help activate the body's relaxation response, lower stress hormone levels, and promote detoxification. Practice deep breathing exercises regularly throughout the day to center yourself and reduce stress.

4. **Nature Walks:** Spending time in nature can have profound benefits for mental and emotional well-being. Take leisurely walks in natural settings, such as parks, forests, or beaches, to connect with the healing power of nature and promote relaxation and inner peace.

5. **Journaling:** Journaling can be a therapeutic practice for processing emotions, reflecting on experiences, and fostering self-awareness during the detoxification process. Set aside time each day to journal about your thoughts, feelings, and experiences, allowing yourself to release stress and gain clarity.

Incorporating Mindfulness into Your Detox Routine

- **Start and end your day with mindfulness:** Begin and end each day with a few minutes of mindfulness practice, whether it's meditation, deep breathing, or simply taking a moment to pause and center yourself.

- **Practice mindful eating:** Slow down and savor each bite of your herbal juices and meals, paying attention to the flavors, textures, and sensations. Mindful eating can enhance digestion, promote satisfaction, and reduce overeating.

- **Stay present in the moment:** Cultivate mindfulness throughout your day by staying present in the moment and fully engaging in each activity. Whether you're preparing herbal juices, exercising, or spending time with loved ones, bring your full attention to the present moment.

Conclusion

Incorporating mindfulness and relaxation techniques into your detoxification routine can enhance the effectiveness of your detox efforts and promote overall well-being. By cultivating a sense of calm and presence, you can support your body's natural detoxification processes, reduce stress levels, and nurture your mind, body, and spirit. Experiment with different mindfulness practices to discover what resonates with you and incorporate them into your daily routine. Stay tuned for more insights and inspiration on your herbal juicing journey. Keep juicing and thriving!

CHAPTER TEN

Day 7: Reflecting on Your Detox Journey and Transitioning to a Healthy Lifestyle

Congratulations on reaching the final day of your herbal juicing journey! As you conclude your detoxification process, it's essential to take time for reflection, celebrate your achievements, and plan for a smooth transition to a healthy and sustainable lifestyle. In today's guide, we'll explore the importance of reflection, strategies for transitioning to a healthy lifestyle, and tips for maintaining the benefits of your detox journey.

Reflecting on Your Detox Journey

Take a moment to reflect on your detox journey and acknowledge your accomplishments along the way. Consider the following questions:

- What were your motivations for embarking on this detox journey?

- What were the highlights of your experience?

- Did you encounter any challenges or obstacles, and how did you overcome them?

- What did you learn about yourself, your body, and your relationship with food during the detox process?

- How do you feel physically, mentally, and emotionally as you conclude your detox journey?

Transitioning to a Healthy Lifestyle

As you transition out of your detox phase, focus on incorporating healthy habits and practices into your daily life to maintain the benefits of your detox journey. Consider the following strategies:

1. **Gradual Reintroduction of Foods:** Slowly reintroduce solid foods into your diet, starting with easily digestible foods such as fruits, vegetables, whole grains, and lean proteins. Pay attention to how your body responds to different foods and make adjustments accordingly.

2. **Balanced Nutrition:** Continue to prioritize nutrient-dense foods, including plenty of fruits, vegetables, whole grains, lean proteins, and healthy fats, in your daily meals and snacks. Aim for a balanced diet that provides essential vitamins, minerals, antioxidants, and macronutrients to support overall health and well-being.

3. **Regular Physical Activity:** Incorporate regular exercise into your routine to support cardiovascular health, strengthen muscles, and maintain flexibility and mobility. Choose activities that you enjoy, whether it's walking, jogging, cycling, swimming, yoga, or strength training, and aim for at

least 30 minutes of moderate-intensity exercise most days of the week.

4. **Hydration:** Continue to prioritize hydration by drinking plenty of water throughout the day. Aim for at least 8-10 cups of water per day, and adjust your fluid intake based on factors such as climate, physical activity level, and individual hydration needs.

5. **Stress Management:** Incorporate stress management techniques such as meditation, deep breathing exercises, yoga, tai chi, or journaling into your daily routine to promote relaxation, reduce stress levels, and support overall well-being.

Maintaining the Benefits of Your Detox Journey

To maintain the benefits of your detox journey in the long term, consider the following tips:

- **Practice Mindful Eating:** Continue to practice mindful eating by paying attention to hunger and fullness cues, savoring each bite, and choosing nourishing foods that support your health goals.

- **Stay Connected:** Stay connected with your support network, whether it's friends, family, or online communities, to share your experiences, seek advice, and stay motivated on your wellness journey.

- **Set Realistic Goals:** Set realistic and achievable goals for your health and wellness journey, and celebrate your progress along the way. Focus on making small, sustainable changes that align with your values and priorities.

Conclusion

As you conclude your detox journey and transition to a healthy lifestyle, take time to reflect on your experiences, celebrate your achievements, and set intentions for the future. By incorporating healthy habits, practicing self-care, and staying connected with your goals, you can maintain the benefits of your detox journey and continue to thrive in all aspects of your life. Remember that wellness is a journey, not a destination, and every step you take toward a healthier lifestyle is a step in the right direction. Keep juicing, stay mindful, and embrace the journey ahead with positivity and determination. Here's to your health and well-being!

SOME VITAL HERBAL REMEDIES YOU NEED TO KNOW

Red Clover:

Definition: Red clover, scientifically known as Trifolium pratense, is a flowering plant belonging to the legume family. It's native to Europe, Western Asia, and Northwest Africa but has been naturalized in many other regions. Red clover has been used in traditional medicine for various purposes, including its potential to support women's health and menopausal symptoms.

Ingredients: Red clover contains several bioactive compounds, including isoflavones (such as genistein and daidzein), flavonoids, and phytoestrogens. These compounds are believed to contribute to the herb's medicinal properties, including its potential as a hormone-balancing agent and its ability to support cardiovascular health.

How to Prepare: Red clover is typically prepared and consumed as an herbal tea or tincture. To make tea, dried red clover flowers are steeped in hot water for several minutes before being strained and consumed. Tinctures are prepared by steeping the flowers in alcohol or vinegar to extract their active compounds.

Dosage: The appropriate dosage of red clover can vary depending on factors such as age, health status, and the specific preparation being used. It's important to follow the recommended dosage on the product label or consult with a qualified herbalist or healthcare professional for personalized guidance.

How to Use: Red clover tea or tincture is typically taken orally. It's important to use red clover products as directed and to discontinue use if any adverse effects occur.

Side Effects: Red clover is generally considered safe for most people when used in moderate amounts. However, some individuals may experience allergic reactions or digestive upset. It may also interact with certain medications or have adverse effects in individuals with certain health conditions. It's important to use red clover under the guidance of a healthcare professional and to discontinue use if any adverse effects occur.

Red Raspberry:

Definition: Red raspberry, scientifically known as Rubus idaeus, is a species of raspberry native to Europe and northern Asia. It's widely cultivated for its delicious berries and has been used in traditional medicine for various purposes, including its potential to support women's health during pregnancy and childbirth.

Ingredients: Red raspberry contains several bioactive compounds, including flavonoids, ellagic acid, anthocyanins, and vitamin C. These compounds are believed to contribute to the herb's medicinal properties, including its potential as an antioxidant, anti-inflammatory, and uterine tonic.

How to Prepare: Red raspberry leaf is typically prepared and consumed as an herbal tea or infusion. To make tea, dried red raspberry leaves are steeped in hot water for several minutes before being strained and consumed.

Dosage: The appropriate dosage of red raspberry leaf can vary depending on factors such as age, health status, and the specific preparation being used. It's important to follow the recommended dosage on the product label or consult with a qualified herbalist or healthcare professional for personalized guidance.

How to Use: Red raspberry leaf tea is typically taken orally. It's often recommended for pregnant individuals in the later stages of pregnancy to support uterine health and prepare for childbirth. It's important to use red raspberry leaf products as directed and to discontinue use if any adverse effects occur.

Side Effects: Red raspberry leaf is generally considered safe for most people when used in moderate amounts. However, some individuals may experience allergic reactions or digestive upset. Pregnant individuals should consult with a healthcare professional before using red raspberry leaf, especially if they have any underlying health conditions or are taking medications. It's important to use red raspberry leaf under the guidance of a healthcare professional and to discontinue use if any adverse effects occur.

Tila:

Definition: Tila, also known as linden flower or lime blossom, refers to the flowers of the Tilia genus, primarily Tilia europaea and Tilia cordata. These trees are native to Europe, but they are also cultivated in other regions for their fragrant and medicinal flowers.

Ingredients: Tila flowers contain various bioactive compounds, including flavonoids, phenolic acids, and volatile oils. These compounds are believed to contribute to the herb's medicinal properties, including its potential as a mild sedative, anxiolytic, and anti-inflammatory agent.

How to Prepare: Tila flowers are typically prepared and consumed as an herbal tea or infusion. To make tea, dried tila flowers are steeped in hot water for several minutes before being strained and consumed.

Dosage: The appropriate dosage of tila can vary depending on factors such as age, health status, and the specific preparation being used. It's important to follow the recommended dosage on the product label or consult with a qualified herbalist or healthcare professional for personalized guidance.

How to Use: Tila tea is typically taken orally. It's often consumed in the evening as a calming bedtime beverage or during times of stress or anxiety. It's important to use tila products as directed and to discontinue use if any adverse effects occur.

Side Effects: Tila is generally considered safe for most people when used in moderate amounts. However, some individuals may experience allergic reactions or digestive upset. It may also interact with certain medications or have adverse effects in individuals with certain health conditions. It's important to use tila under the guidance of a healthcare professional and to discontinue use if any adverse effects occur.

Valerian:

Definition: Valerian, scientifically known as Valeriana officinalis, is a perennial flowering plant native to Europe and Asia. It has been used for centuries in traditional medicine for its potential calming and sedative effects.

Ingredients: Valerian root contains several bioactive compounds, including valerenic acid, valepotriates, and volatile oils. These compounds are believed to contribute to the herb's medicinal properties, including its potential as a sedative, anxiolytic, and sleep aid.

How to Prepare: Valerian root is typically prepared and consumed as an herbal tea, tincture, or capsule. To make tea, dried valerian root is steeped in hot water for several minutes before being strained and consumed. Tinctures are prepared by steeping the root in alcohol or vinegar to extract its active compounds.

Dosage: The appropriate dosage of valerian can vary depending on factors such as age, health status, and the specific preparation being used. It's important to follow the recommended dosage on the product label or consult with a qualified herbalist or healthcare professional for personalized guidance.

How to Use: Valerian tea, tincture, or capsules are typically taken orally. It's often consumed in the evening as a sleep aid or during times of stress or anxiety. It's important to use valerian products as directed and to discontinue use if any adverse effects occur.

Side Effects: Valerian is generally considered safe for most people when used in moderate amounts. However, some individuals may experience mild side effects such as drowsiness, headache, or gastrointestinal upset. It may also interact with certain medications or have adverse effects in individuals with certain health conditions. It's important to use valerian under the guidance of a healthcare professional and to discontinue use if any adverse effects occur.

Wild Cherry Bark:

Definition: Wild cherry bark, scientifically known as Prunus serotina, is the bark obtained from the black cherry tree native to North America. It has been used traditionally in Native American and folk medicine for its potential health benefits, particularly for respiratory and digestive issues.

Ingredients: Wild cherry bark contains various bioactive compounds, including cyanogenic glycosides (such as prunasin and amygdalin), flavonoids, and phenolic acids. These compounds are believed to contribute to the herb's medicinal properties, including its potential as an expectorant, cough suppressant, and mild sedative.

How to Prepare: Wild cherry bark is typically prepared and consumed as an herbal tea, decoction, or syrup. To make tea, dried wild cherry bark is steeped in hot water for several minutes before being strained and consumed. Decoctions involve boiling the bark in water to extract its active compounds, while syrups are made by simmering the bark with sugar or honey to create a thick, sweet liquid.

Dosage: The appropriate dosage of wild cherry bark can vary depending on factors such as age, health status, and the specific preparation being used. It's important to follow the recommended dosage on the product label or consult with a qualified herbalist or healthcare professional for personalized guidance.

How to Use: Wild cherry bark tea, decoction, or syrup is typically taken orally. It's often consumed to soothe coughs, sore throats, and other respiratory symptoms. It's important to use wild cherry bark products as directed and to discontinue use if any adverse effects occur.

Side Effects: Wild cherry bark is generally considered safe for most people when used in moderate amounts. However, it contains cyanogenic glycosides, which can release cyanide in the body when metabolized. While the risk of cyanide poisoning from consuming wild cherry bark is low when used appropriately, excessive intake or prolonged use may lead to adverse effects. It's important to use wild cherry bark under the guidance of a healthcare professional and to discontinue use if any adverse effects occur.

Yellowdock:

Definition: Yellowdock, scientifically known as Rumex crispus, is a perennial flowering plant native to Europe and western Asia but is also found in North America. It has a long history of use in traditional medicine, particularly among Indigenous peoples, for its potential health benefits.

Ingredients: Yellowdock root contains various bioactive compounds, including anthraquinone glycosides (such as emodin and chrysophanol), tannins, and vitamins (including vitamin A and vitamin C). These compounds are believed to contribute to the herb's medicinal properties, including its potential as a laxative, blood cleanser, and liver tonic.

How to Prepare: Yellowdock root is typically prepared and consumed as an herbal tea, tincture, or capsule. To make tea, dried yellowdock root is steeped in hot water for several minutes before being strained and consumed. Tinctures are prepared by steeping the root in alcohol or vinegar to extract its active compounds.

Dosage: The appropriate dosage of yellowdock can vary depending on factors such as age, health status, and the specific preparation being used. It's important to follow the recommended dosage on the product label or consult with a qualified herbalist or healthcare professional for personalized guidance.

How to Use: Yellowdock tea, tincture, or capsules are typically taken orally. It's often consumed to support digestion, promote bowel regularity, and cleanse the blood. It's important to use yellowdock products as directed and to discontinue use if any adverse effects occur.

Side Effects: Yellowdock is generally considered safe for most people when used in moderate amounts. However, some individuals may experience mild side effects such as gastrointestinal upset or allergic reactions. It may also interact with certain medications or have adverse effects in individuals with certain health conditions. It's important to use yellowdock under the guidance of a healthcare professional and to discontinue use if any adverse effects occur.

Yellowdock Root:

Definition: Yellowdock root, scientifically known as Rumex crispus, is the root of a perennial flowering plant native to Europe and western Asia, also found in North America. It has a long history of use in traditional medicine, particularly among Indigenous peoples, for its potential health benefits.

Ingredients: Yellowdock root contains various bioactive compounds, including anthraquinone glycosides (such as emodin and chrysophanol), tannins, and vitamins (including vitamin A and vitamin C). These compounds are believed to contribute to the herb's medicinal properties, including its potential as a laxative, blood cleanser, and liver tonic.

How to Prepare: Yellowdock root is typically prepared and consumed as an herbal tea, tincture, or capsule. To make tea, dried yellowdock root is steeped in hot water for several minutes before being strained and consumed. Tinctures are prepared by steeping the root in alcohol or vinegar to extract its active compounds.

Dosage: The appropriate dosage of yellowdock root can vary depending on factors such as age, health status, and the specific preparation being used. It's important to follow the recommended dosage on the product label or consult with a qualified herbalist or healthcare professional for personalized guidance.

How to Use: Yellowdock root tea, tincture, or capsules are typically taken orally. It's often consumed to support digestion, promote bowel regularity, and cleanse the blood. It's important to use yellowdock root products as directed and to discontinue use if any adverse effects occur.

Side Effects: Yellowdock root is generally considered safe for most people when used in moderate amounts. However, some individuals may experience mild side effects such as gastrointestinal upset or allergic reactions. It may also interact with certain medications or have adverse effects in individuals with certain health conditions. It's important to use yellowdock root under the guidance of a healthcare professional and to discontinue use if any adverse effects occur.

Agrimony:

Definition: Agrimony, scientifically known as Agrimonia eupatoria, is a perennial herbaceous plant native to Europe, Asia, and North America. It has a long history of use in traditional medicine, particularly in European folk medicine, for its potential health benefits.

Ingredients: Agrimony contains various bioactive compounds, including tannins, flavonoids, phenolic acids, and volatile oils. These compounds are believed to contribute to the herb's medicinal properties, including its potential as an astringent, anti-inflammatory, and digestive aid.

How to Prepare: Agrimony is typically prepared and consumed as an herbal tea, tincture, or poultice. To make tea, dried agrimony leaves and flowers are steeped in hot water for several minutes before being strained and consumed. Tinctures are prepared by steeping the herb in alcohol or vinegar to extract its active compounds.

Dosage: The appropriate dosage of agrimony can vary depending on factors such as age, health status, and the specific preparation being used. It's important to follow the recommended dosage on the product label or consult with a qualified herbalist or healthcare professional for personalized guidance.

How to Use: Agrimony tea, tincture, or poultice is typically taken orally or applied topically. It's often consumed to soothe gastrointestinal issues, such as indigestion and diarrhea, or used externally to treat skin conditions.

Side Effects: Agrimony is generally considered safe for most people when used in moderate amounts. However, some individuals may experience allergic reactions or gastrointestinal upset. It may also interact with certain medications or have adverse effects in individuals with certain health conditions. It's important to use agrimony under the guidance of a healthcare professional and to discontinue use if any adverse effects occur.

Alfalfa:

Definition: Alfalfa, scientifically known as Medicago sativa, is a flowering plant in the pea family native to Asia but cultivated worldwide. It's primarily grown as fodder for livestock, but it has also been used in traditional medicine for its potential health benefits.

Ingredients: Alfalfa contains various bioactive compounds, including vitamins (such as vitamin A, vitamin C, and vitamin K), minerals (including calcium, magnesium, and potassium), amino acids, and phytoestrogens. These compounds are believed to contribute to the herb's medicinal properties, including its potential as a nutritive tonic, diuretic, and hormone balancer.

How to Prepare: Alfalfa is typically consumed as sprouts, herbal tea, or in supplement form (such as capsules or tablets). To make tea, dried alfalfa leaves are steeped in hot water for several minutes before being strained and consumed.

Dosage: The appropriate dosage of alfalfa can vary depending on factors such as age, health status, and the specific preparation being used. It's important to follow the recommended dosage on the product label or consult with a qualified herbalist or healthcare professional for personalized guidance.

How to Use: Alfalfa sprouts, tea, or supplements are typically taken orally. It's often consumed as a dietary supplement to support overall health and well-being, as well as to promote kidney health and hormone balance.

Side Effects: Alfalfa is generally considered safe for most people when consumed in moderate amounts. However, some individuals may experience allergic reactions or digestive upset. It may also interact with certain medications or have adverse effects in individuals with certain health conditions, such as autoimmune diseases or hormone-sensitive conditions. Pregnant or breastfeeding individuals should consult with a healthcare professional before using alfalfa supplements. It's important to use alfalfa under the guidance of a healthcare professional and to discontinue use if any adverse effects occur.

Ashwagandha:

Definition: Ashwagandha, scientifically known as Withaniasomnifera, is a small shrub native to India, the Middle East, and parts of Africa. It has a long history of use in Ayurvedic medicine for its potential health benefits, particularly for its adaptogenic properties.

Ingredients: Ashwagandha root contains various bioactive compounds, including alkaloids (such as withanolides), steroidal lactones, and flavonoids. These compounds are believed to contribute to the herb's medicinal properties, including its potential as an adaptogen, anti-inflammatory, and immune-modulating agent.

How to Prepare: Ashwagandha is typically consumed as a powdered root, herbal tea, tincture, or in supplement form (such as capsules or tablets). To make tea, dried ashwagandha root is steeped in hot water for several minutes before being strained and consumed.

Dosage: The appropriate dosage of ashwagandha can vary depending on factors such as age, health status, and the specific preparation being used. It's important to follow the recommended dosage on the product label or consult with a qualified herbalist or healthcare professional for personalized guidance.

How to Use: Ashwagandha powder, tea, tincture, or supplements are typically taken orally. It's often consumed to support stress management, promote relaxation, and boost overall vitality and well-being.

Side Effects: Ashwagandha is generally considered safe for most people when used in moderate amounts. However, some individuals may experience mild side effects such as gastrointestinal upset or drowsiness. It may also interact with certain medications or have adverse effects in individuals with certain health conditions, such as autoimmune diseases or thyroid disorders. Pregnant or breastfeeding individuals should consult with a healthcare professional before using ashwagandha supplements. It's important to use ashwagandha under the guidance of a healthcare professional and to discontinue use if any adverse effects occur.

Astragalus:

Definition: Astragalus, scientifically known as Astragalus membranaceus, is a flowering plant native to China and Mongolia but also found in other parts of Asia. It has been used for centuries in traditional Chinese medicine for its potential health benefits, particularly for its immune-enhancing properties.

Ingredients: Astragalus root contains various bioactive compounds, including polysaccharides, saponins (such as astragalosides), flavonoids, and amino acids. These compounds are believed to contribute to the herb's medicinal properties, including its potential as an adaptogen, immunomodulator, and anti-inflammatory agent.

How to Prepare: Astragalus is typically consumed as a powdered root, herbal tea, tincture, or in supplement form (such as capsules or tablets). To make tea, dried astragalus root slices are simmered in water for several minutes before being strained and consumed.

Dosage: The appropriate dosage of astragalus can vary depending on factors such as age, health status, and the specific preparation being used. It's important to follow the recommended dosage on the product label or consult with a qualified herbalist or healthcare professional for personalized guidance.

How to Use: Astragalus powder, tea, tincture, or supplements are typically taken orally. It's often consumed to support immune function, promote vitality, and enhance overall well-being.

Side Effects: Astragalus is generally considered safe for most people when used in moderate amounts. However, some individuals may experience mild side effects such as gastrointestinal upset or allergic reactions. It may also interact with certain medications or have adverse effects in individuals with certain health conditions, such as autoimmune diseases or diabetes. Pregnant or breastfeeding individuals should consult with a healthcare professional before using astragalus supplements. It's important to use astragalus under the guidance of a healthcare professional and to discontinue use if any adverse effects occur.

Cat's Claw:

Definition: Cat's claw, scientifically known as Uncaria tomentosa, is a woody vine native to the Amazon rainforest and other parts of Central and South America. It has been used for centuries in traditional medicine by indigenous peoples for its potential health benefits.

Ingredients: Cat's claw contains various bioactive compounds, including alkaloids (such as oxindole alkaloids and quinovic acid glycosides), polyphenols, and other phytochemicals. These compounds are believed to contribute to the herb's medicinal properties, including its potential as an immune enhancer, anti-inflammatory, and antioxidant.

How to Prepare: Cat's claw is typically consumed as an herbal tea, tincture, or in supplement form (such as capsules or tablets). To make tea, dried cat's claw bark or leaves are steeped in hot water for several minutes before being strained and consumed.

Dosage: The appropriate dosage of cat's claw can vary depending on factors such as age, health status, and the specific preparation being used. It's important to follow the recommended dosage on the product label or consult with a qualified herbalist or healthcare professional for personalized guidance.

How to Use: Cat's claw tea, tincture, or supplements are typically taken orally. It's often used to support immune function, reduce inflammation, and promote overall well-being.

Side Effects: Cat's claw is generally considered safe for most people when used in moderate amounts. However, some individuals may experience mild side effects such as gastrointestinal upset or allergic reactions. It may also interact with certain medications or have adverse effects in individuals with certain health conditions, such as autoimmune diseases or bleeding disorders. Pregnant or breastfeeding individuals should consult with a healthcare professional before using cat's claw supplements. It's important to use cat's claw under the guidance of a healthcare professional and to discontinue use if any adverse effects occur.

Chickweed:

Definition: Chickweed, scientifically known as Stellaria media, is an annual herbaceous plant native to Europe but naturalized in many other parts of the world. It's often considered a common weed but has been used historically in traditional medicine for its potential health benefits.

Ingredients: Chickweed contains various bioactive compounds, including flavonoids, saponins, mucilage, and vitamins (such as vitamin C). These compounds are believed to contribute to the herb's medicinal properties, including its potential as a demulcent, anti-inflammatory, and mild diuretic.

How to Prepare: Chickweed is typically consumed as an herbal tea, infusion, or in fresh salads. To make tea, dried chickweed leaves and flowers are steeped in hot water for several minutes before being strained and consumed. It can also be used topically as a poultice or infused oil for skin conditions.

Dosage: The appropriate dosage of chickweed can vary depending on factors such as age, health status, and the specific preparation being used. It's important to follow the recommended dosage on the product label or consult with a qualified herbalist or healthcare professional for personalized guidance.

How to Use: Chickweed tea, infusion, or fresh leaves are typically taken orally. It's often used to soothe inflammation, support digestion, and promote overall well-being. Topically, chickweed can be applied to the skin to alleviate itching, irritation, or minor wounds.

Side Effects: Chickweed is generally considered safe for most people when consumed in moderate amounts. However, some individuals may experience allergic reactions or gastrointestinal upset. It may also interact with certain medications or have adverse effects in individuals with certain health conditions. Pregnant or breastfeeding individuals should consult with a healthcare professional before using chickweed supplements. It's important to use chickweed under the guidance of a healthcare professional and to discontinue use if any adverse effects occur.

Cleavers:

Definition: Cleavers, scientifically known as Galium aparine, is a herbaceous annual plant native to Europe, North America, Asia, and Australia. It has a long history of use in traditional medicine for its potential health benefits.

Ingredients: Cleavers contains various bioactive compounds, including iridoid glycosides, flavonoids, tannins, and mucilage. These compounds are believed to contribute to the herb's medicinal properties, including its potential as a diuretic, lymphatic tonic, and mild astringent.

How to Prepare: Cleavers is typically consumed as an herbal tea, infusion, or in fresh salads. To make tea, dried cleavers leaves and stems are steeped in hot water for several minutes before being strained and consumed. It can also be used topically as a poultice or infused oil for skin conditions.

Dosage: The appropriate dosage of cleavers can vary depending on factors such as age, health status, and the specific preparation being used. It's important to follow the recommended dosage on the product label or consult with a qualified herbalist or healthcare professional for personalized guidance.

How to Use: Cleavers tea, infusion, or fresh leaves are typically taken orally. It's often used to support lymphatic drainage, promote urinary tract health, and soothe inflammation. Topically, cleavers can be applied to the skin to alleviate itching, irritation, or minor wounds.

Side Effects: Cleavers is generally considered safe for most people when consumed in moderate amounts. However, some individuals may experience allergic reactions or gastrointestinal upset. It may also interact with certain medications or have adverse effects in individuals with certain health conditions. Pregnant or breastfeeding individuals should consult with a healthcare professional before using cleavers supplements. It's important to use cleavers under the guidance of a healthcare professional and to discontinue use if any adverse effects occur.

Eucalyptus:

Definition: Eucalyptus refers to a genus of flowering trees and shrubs, primarily native to Australia but also found in other parts of the world. Eucalyptus essential oil, extracted from the leaves of certain species, has a long history of use in traditional medicine for its potential health benefits.

Ingredients: Eucalyptus essential oil contains various bioactive compounds, including eucalyptol (cineole), terpenes, and flavonoids. These compounds are believed to contribute to the oil's medicinal properties, including its potential as an expectorant, decongestant, antiseptic, and anti-inflammatory.

How to Prepare: Eucalyptus essential oil can be used in aromatherapy, diffused in the air, or diluted and applied topically to the skin. It can also be added to steam inhalations or chest rubs to help relieve respiratory symptoms.

Dosage: The appropriate dosage of eucalyptus essential oil can vary depending on factors such as age, health status, and the specific application being used. It's important to follow the recommended dosage on the product label or consult with a qualified aromatherapist or healthcare professional for personalized guidance.

How to Use: Eucalyptus essential oil can be used aromatically, topically, or internally, depending on the intended application. It's often used to alleviate respiratory congestion, soothe sore muscles, promote relaxation, and support overall well-being.

Side Effects: Eucalyptus essential oil is generally considered safe for most people when used appropriately. However, it can be toxic if ingested in large amounts and should not be applied directly to the skin without proper dilution. Some individuals may experience allergic reactions or respiratory irritation when exposed to eucalyptus oil. It's important to use eucalyptus oil with caution, especially around children and pets. Pregnant or breastfeeding individuals should consult with a healthcare professional before using eucalyptus oil. If any adverse effects occur, discontinue use and seek medical attention.

Feverfew:

Definition: Feverfew, scientifically known as Tanacetum parthenium, is a perennial herb native to Europe but also found in other parts of the world. It has a long history of use in traditional medicine, particularly in European folk medicine, for its potential health benefits.

Ingredients: Feverfew contains various bioactive compounds, including sesquiterpene lactones (such as parthenolide), flavonoids, and volatile oils. These compounds are believed to contribute to the herb's medicinal properties, including its potential as an anti-inflammatory, analgesic, and migraine prophylactic.

How to Prepare: Feverfew is typically consumed as an herbal tea, tincture, or in supplement form (such as capsules or tablets). To make tea, dried feverfew leaves and flowers are steeped in hot water for several minutes before being strained and consumed.

Dosage: The appropriate dosage of feverfew can vary depending on factors such as age, health status, and the specific preparation being used. It's important to follow the recommended dosage on the product label or consult with a qualified herbalist or healthcare professional for personalized guidance.

How to Use: Feverfew tea, tincture, or supplements are typically taken orally. It's often used to alleviate headaches, including migraines, and to support overall well-being.

Side Effects: Feverfew is generally considered safe for most people when used in moderate amounts. However, some individuals may experience mild side effects such as gastrointestinal upset or allergic reactions. It may also interact with certain medications or have adverse effects in individuals with certain health conditions, such as bleeding disorders or pregnancy. It's important to use feverfew under the guidance of a healthcare professional and to discontinue use if any adverse effects occur.

Ginseng:

Definition: Ginseng refers to several species of perennial plants belonging to the Panax genus, including Panax ginseng (Asian ginseng) and Panax quinquefolius (American ginseng). Ginseng has been used for centuries in traditional medicine, particularly in East Asia, for its potential health benefits.

Ingredients: Ginseng root contains various bioactive compounds, including ginsenosides, polysaccharides, and peptides. These compounds are believed to contribute to the herb's medicinal properties, including its potential as an adaptogen, immune enhancer, and cognitive booster.

How to Prepare: Ginseng is typically consumed as a powdered root, herbal tea, tincture, or in supplement form (such as capsules or tablets). To make tea, dried ginseng root slices are simmered in water for several minutes before being strained and consumed.

Dosage: The appropriate dosage of ginseng can vary depending on factors such as age, health status, and the specific preparation being used. It's important to follow the recommended dosage on the product label or consult with a qualified herbalist or healthcare professional for personalized guidance.

How to Use: Ginseng powder, tea, tincture, or supplements are typically taken orally. It's often used to support energy levels, enhance cognitive function, and promote overall well-being.

Side Effects: Ginseng is generally considered safe for most people when used in moderate amounts. However, some individuals may experience mild side effects such as insomnia, gastrointestinal upset, or headaches. It may also interact with certain medications or have adverse effects in individuals with certain health conditions, such as high blood pressure or diabetes. Pregnant or breastfeeding individuals should consult with a healthcare professional before using ginseng supplements. It's important to use ginseng under the guidance of a healthcare professional and to discontinue use if any adverse effects occur.

Goldenseal:

Definition: Goldenseal, scientifically known as Hydrastis canadensis, is a perennial herb native to North America. It has a long history of use in traditional Native American medicine and later in folk medicine for its potential health benefits.

Ingredients: Goldenseal root contains various bioactive compounds, including alkaloids (such as berberine and hydrastine), flavonoids, and volatile oils. These compounds are believed to contribute to the herb's medicinal properties, including its potential as an antimicrobial, anti-inflammatory, and immune enhancer.

How to Prepare: Goldenseal is typically consumed as an herbal tea, tincture, or in supplement form (such as capsules or tablets). To make tea, dried goldenseal root or leaves are steeped in hot water for several minutes before being strained and consumed.

Dosage: The appropriate dosage of goldenseal can vary depending on factors such as age, health status, and the specific preparation being used. It's important to follow the recommended dosage on the product label or consult with a qualified herbalist or healthcare professional for personalized guidance.

How to Use: Goldenseal tea, tincture, or supplements are typically taken orally. It's often used to support immune function, promote digestive health, and soothe inflammation.

Side Effects: Goldenseal is generally considered safe for most people when used in moderate amounts. However, some individuals may experience mild side effects such as gastrointestinal upset or allergic reactions. It may also interact with certain medications or have adverse effects in individuals with certain health conditions, such as high blood pressure or pregnancy. It's important to use goldenseal under the guidance of a healthcare professional and to discontinue use if any adverse effects occur.

Hops:

Definition: Hops, scientifically known as Humulus lupulus, is a perennial climbing vine native to Europe, Asia, and North America. It is primarily known for its use in brewing beer but has also been used historically in traditional medicine for its potential health benefits.

Ingredients: Hops flowers contain various bioactive compounds, including bitter acids (such as humulone and lupulone), essential oils, flavonoids, and polyphenols. These compounds are believed to contribute to the herb's medicinal properties, including its potential as a sedative, relaxant, and digestive aid.

How to Prepare: Hops is typically consumed as an herbal tea, tincture, or in supplement form (such as capsules or tablets). To make tea, dried hops flowers are steeped in hot water for several minutes before being strained and consumed.

Dosage: The appropriate dosage of hops can vary depending on factors such as age, health status, and the specific preparation being used. It's important to follow the recommended dosage on the product label or consult with a qualified herbalist or healthcare professional for personalized guidance.

How to Use: Hops tea, tincture, or supplements are typically taken orally. It's often used to promote relaxation, relieve anxiety, and support sleep.

Side Effects: Hops is generally considered safe for most people when used in moderate amounts. However, some individuals may experience mild side effects such as drowsiness, gastrointestinal upset, or allergic reactions. It may also interact with certain medications or have adverse effects in individuals with certain health conditions, such as depression or hormone-sensitive conditions. It's important to use hops under the guidance of a healthcare professional and to discontinue use if any adverse effects occur.

Kelp:

Definition: Kelp refers to several species of large brown algae belonging to the Laminariales order. It is commonly found in underwater forests along rocky coastlines around the world. Kelp has been used for centuries in various cultures, particularly in East Asia, for its nutritional and medicinal properties.

Ingredients: Kelp is rich In various nutrients, including iodine, vitamins (such as vitamin K, vitamin C, and B vitamins), minerals (including calcium, magnesium, and potassium), antioxidants, and fiber. These nutrients are believed to contribute to the seaweed's potential health benefits, including its role in thyroid function, bone health, and immune support.

How to Prepare: Kelp is typically consumed dried, powdered, or in supplement form (such as capsules or tablets). It can also be used in cooking, particularly in soups, salads, and stir-fries. Kelp supplements are available in various forms, including powdered extracts, tablets, and liquid extracts.

Dosage: The appropriate dosage of kelp can vary depending on factors such as age, health status, and the specific preparation being used. It's important to follow the recommended dosage on the product label or consult with a qualified healthcare professional for personalized guidance.

How to Use: Kelp supplements are typically taken orally with water. They can be consumed as part of a daily nutritional regimen to support overall health and well-being. Kelp can also be incorporated into recipes as a flavorful and nutritious ingredient.

Side Effects: While kelp is generally considered safe for most people when consumed in moderate amounts, excessive intake of iodine-rich foods or supplements, including kelp, can lead to thyroid dysfunction or iodine toxicity. Some individuals may also be allergic to seaweed and experience allergic reactions. Pregnant or breastfeeding individuals should consult with a healthcare professional before using kelp supplements. It's important to use kelp under the guidance of a healthcare professional and to discontinue use if any adverse effects occur.

Black Cohosh:

Definition: Black cohosh, scientifically known as Actaea racemosa (formerly Cimicifuga racemosa), is a perennial herb native to North America. It has a long history of use in traditional Native American medicine and later in folk medicine for its potential health benefits, particularly for women's health.

Ingredients: Black cohosh root contains various bioactive compounds, including triterpene glycosides (such as actein and cimicifugoside), phenolic acids, and flavonoids. These compounds are believed to contribute to the herb's medicinal properties, including its potential as a hormone-balancing agent and its ability to relieve menopausal symptoms.

How to Prepare: Black cohosh is typically consumed as a powdered root, herbal tea, tincture, or in supplement form (such as capsules or tablets). To make tea, dried black cohosh root is steeped in hot water for several minutes before being strained and consumed.

Dosage: The appropriate dosage of black cohosh can vary depending on factors such as age, health status, and the specific preparation being used. It's important to follow the recommended dosage on the product label or consult with a qualified herbalist or healthcare professional for personalized guidance.

How to Use: Black cohosh powder, tea, tincture, or supplements are typically taken orally. It's often used by women to support hormonal balance, relieve menopausal symptoms such as hot flashes and night sweats, and promote overall well-being.

Side Effects: Black cohosh is generally considered safe for most people when used in moderate amounts. However, some individuals may experience mild side effects such as gastrointestinal upset or allergic reactions. It may also interact with certain medications or have adverse effects in individuals with certain health conditions, such as liver disease or hormone-sensitive conditions. Pregnant or breastfeeding individuals should consult with a healthcare professional before using black cohosh supplements. It's important to use black cohosh under the guidance of a healthcare professional and to discontinue use if any adverse effects occur.

Blessed Thistle:

Definition: Blessed thistle, scientifically known as Cnicusbenedictus, is an annual or biennial herb native to the Mediterranean region but also found in other parts of Europe, Asia, and North Africa. It has been used historically in traditional medicine for its potential health benefits, particularly for digestive and liver health.

Ingredients: Blessed thistle contains various bioactive compounds, including sesquiterpene lactones (such as cnicin), flavonoids, tannins, and essential oils. These compounds are believed to contribute to the herb's medicinal properties, including its potential as a digestive tonic, appetite stimulant, and liver tonic.

How to Prepare: Blessed thistle is typically consumed as an herbal tea, tincture, or in supplement form (such as capsules or tablets). To make tea, dried blessed thistle leaves and flowers are steeped in hot water for several minutes before being strained and consumed.

Dosage: The appropriate dosage of blessed thistle can vary depending on factors such as age, health status, and the specific preparation being used. It's important to follow the recommended dosage on the product label or consult with a qualified herbalist or healthcare professional for personalized guidance.

How to Use: Blessed thistle tea, tincture, or supplements are typically taken orally. It's often used to support digestion, stimulate appetite, and promote liver health.

Side Effects: Blessed thistle is generally considered safe for most people when used in moderate amounts. However, some individuals may experience mild side effects such as gastrointestinal upset or allergic reactions. It may also interact with certain medications or have adverse effects in individuals with certain health conditions, such as hormone-sensitive conditions or bleeding disorders. Pregnant or breastfeeding individuals should consult with a healthcare professional before using blessed thistle supplements. It's important to use blessed thistle under the guidance of a healthcare professional and to discontinue use if any adverse effects occur.

Rhubarb:

Definition: Rhubarb, scientifically known as Rheum rhabarbarum, is a perennial plant cultivated for its edible stalks. While primarily used in culinary applications, rhubarb has also been utilized in traditional medicine for its potential health benefits, particularly for digestive health.

Ingredients: Rhubarb stalks contain various bioactive compounds, including anthraquinones (such as emodin and rhein), fiber, vitamins (such as vitamin K), and minerals (including calcium and potassium). These compounds are believed to contribute to the herb's medicinal properties, including its potential as a laxative and digestive aid.

How to Prepare: Rhubarb stalks are typically cooked before consumption, as the raw stalks are very tart and can be unpleasant to eat. They are often used in pies, crisps, jams, sauces, and other desserts, as well as in savory dishes. Rhubarb can also be used to make compotes, jams, and preserves.

Dosage: There is no specific dosage for rhubarb in culinary applications, as it is used as a food rather than a medicinal herb. However, when used for its potential laxative effects, it's important to consume rhubarb in moderation to avoid gastrointestinal upset.

How to Use: Rhubarb stalks can be chopped and cooked in various dishes, including pies, sauces, and jams. It's important to remove and discard the leaves, as they contain toxic compounds. When using rhubarb for its potential laxative effects, it's typically consumed as part of a cooked dish or in the form of a rhubarb-based herbal remedy.

Side Effects: Rhubarb stalks are generally safe for most people when consumed in moderate amounts as part of a balanced diet. However, excessive intake may lead to digestive upset or adverse effects due to the presence of oxalic acid, which can bind to calcium and form kidney stones in susceptible individuals. It's important to use rhubarb in moderation and to consult with a healthcare professional if you have any concerns or underlying health conditions.

Sarsaparilla:

Definition: Sarsaparilla refers to several species of plants belonging to the Smilax genus, including Smilax regelii and Smilax officinalis. It has been used historically in traditional medicine for its potential health benefits, particularly for its purported detoxifying and anti-inflammatory properties.

Ingredients: Sarsaparilla contains various bioactive compounds, including saponins (such as sarsaponin and smilagenin), flavonoids, phenolic acids, and sterols. These compounds are believed to contribute to the herb's medicinal properties, including its potential as a diuretic, blood purifier, and anti-inflammatory agent.

How to Prepare: Sarsaparilla root is typically prepared and consumed as an herbal tea, decoction, or tincture. To make tea, dried sarsaparilla root is steeped in hot water for several minutes before being strained and consumed. Decoctions involve boiling the root in water to extract its active compounds, while tinctures are prepared by steeping the root in alcohol or vinegar.

Dosage: The appropriate dosage of sarsaparilla can vary depending on factors such as age, health status, and the specific preparation being used. It's important to follow the recommended dosage on the product label or consult with a qualified herbalist or healthcare professional for personalized guidance.

How to Use: Sarsaparilla tea or tincture is typically taken orally. It's important to use sarsaparilla products as directed and to discontinue use if any adverse effects occur.

Side Effects: Sarsaparilla is generally considered safe for most people when used in moderate amounts. However, some individuals may experience allergic reactions or digestive upset. It may also interact with certain medications or have adverse effects in individuals with certain health conditions. It's important to use sarsaparilla under the guidance of a healthcare professional and to discontinue use if any adverse effects occur.

THE END